EFFECTIVE WORKOUT STRATEGIES FOR SENIORS

Understanding Fitness Needs And Choosing The Right Type Of Exercises

Dr. Abigail Lucas

1

TABLE OF CONTENTS

Introduction
A. Importance of exercise for seniors' overall well-being
B. Challenges faced by seniors in maintaining fitness levels
C. Purpose of the guide: providing practical and effective workout strategies tailored for seniors

II. Understanding Senior Fitness Needs
A. Physiological changes associated with aging
B. Common health concerns and their impact on exercise
C. Benefits of age-appropriate workouts, including improved strength, balance, and flexibility

III. Preparing for Safe Exercise
A. Consultation with healthcare professionals
before starting any workout routine
B. Importance of warm-up and cool-down exercises
C. Choosing suitable workout attire and footwear
for safety and comfort

IV. Low-Impact and Senior-Friendly Exercises
A. Gentle cardiovascular exercises (e.g., walking,
swimming)
B. Strength training with light weights or resistance
bands
C. Balance and flexibility exercises (e.g., yoga, tai
chi)
D. Chair exercises and seated workouts for seniors
with limited mobility

V. Designing Personalized Workout Plans
A. Assessing individual fitness levels and setting
realistic goals
B. Creating customized workout routines based on
seniors' abilities and preferences
C. Adapting exercises for seniors with specific
health conditions or physical limitations

VI. Motivation and Consistency
A. Setting achievable goals and tracking progress

B. Incorporating social activities and group exercises for motivation
C. Overcoming common obstacles and staying consistent with workouts

VII. Nutrition and Recovery
A. Importance of a balanced diet and hydration for seniors
B. Rest and recovery techniques to prevent fatigue and injuries
C. Incorporating proper nutrition to support exercise and promote muscle recovery

VIII. Dealing with Challenges
A. Addressing fear and anxiety related to exercise
B. Coping with pain, discomfort, or fatigue during workouts
C. Seeking support and encouragement from family, friends, or support groups

IX. Special Considerations
A. Exercise guidelines for seniors with specific health conditions (e.g., arthritis, osteoporosis)
B. Senior-friendly modifications for home workouts and gym environments
C. Travel-friendly exercises for seniors who are frequently on the move

X. Conclusion
A. Recap of key points and takeaways
B. Encouragement for seniors to embrace the benefits of regular exercise
C. Resources and references for further information and support

INTRODUCTION

Once in the peaceful town of Harmony Grove, a group of seniors decided it was never too late to embark on a journey toward better health and fitness. Led by their enthusiastic community center director, Mrs. Thompson, they embarked on a mission to discover effective workout strategies tailored just for them.

In the heart of Harmony Grove, at the bright and welcoming community center, a diverse group of seniors gathered one sunny morning. Among them were Mr. and Mrs. Johnson, a couple in their 70s eager to regain their vitality; Mrs. Lewis, an 80-year-old with a passion for dance; and Mr. Patel, a sprightly 65-year-old determined to improve his balance.

Under Mrs. Thompson's guidance, they started with gentle warm-up exercises, stretching their arms and legs, and taking deep breaths of fresh air. Mrs. Thompson, armed with a wealth of knowledge, introduced them to low-impact activities like walking and swimming, ensuring everyone could participate at their own pace.

For those seeking to improve their strength, Mrs. Thompson introduced resistance bands and light weights, emphasizing proper techniques to avoid strain. Mrs. Lewis, with her love for dancing, found joy in senior-friendly dance routines that not only kept her active but also lifted her spirits.

In a corner of the community center, Mr. Patel, who initially struggled with balance, discovered the wonders of yoga and tai chi. With patience and practice, he soon found himself more stable and confident on his feet, his determination paying off.

As the weeks passed, the seniors not only grew physically stronger but also formed a close-knit community. They motivated each other, celebrated small victories, and supported those who faced challenges. With consistent guidance and encouragement from Mrs. Thompson, they embraced the importance of balanced nutrition, ensuring their bodies were well-fueled for their newfound activities.

Every day, the community center echoed with laughter, determination, and the sound of cheerful music accompanying the seniors' exercises. They learned that age was just a number, and with the right strategies, anyone could lead an active and fulfilling life.

One day, as the sun set over Harmony Grove, the seniors gathered for a small celebration. They shared stories of their progress, the hurdles they overcame, and the friendships they had forged. Mrs. Thompson stood proudly among them, her heart swelling with happiness.

In Harmony Grove, the tale of these resilient seniors became an inspiration. The message was clear: no matter their age, with effective workout strategies, dedication, and a supportive community, anyone could embark on a journey toward better health. And so, the story of the seniors of Harmony Grove served as a beacon of hope, reminding everyone that it's never too late for a new beginning.

Importance of exercise for seniors' overall well-being

Exercise plays a crucial role in promoting the overall well-being of seniors in various ways. Here are the key reasons why regular physical activity is important for seniors:

Maintaining Physical Health: Regular exercise helps seniors maintain a healthy weight, improve cardiovascular health, and strengthen muscles and bones. It can also enhance flexibility and balance, reducing the risk of falls and fractures, which are common concerns for older adults.

Managing Chronic Conditions: Exercise is instrumental in managing and preventing chronic conditions such as heart disease, diabetes, and arthritis. It can help control blood pressure, lower cholesterol levels, and regulate blood sugar, thereby improving the quality of life for seniors living with these conditions.

Boosting Mental Health: Physical activity releases endorphins, the body's natural stress relievers, which can alleviate symptoms of depression and anxiety. Regular exercise is also associated with improved cognitive function and reduced risk of dementia in seniors.

Enhancing Mobility and Independence: By improving strength, balance, and flexibility, exercise enables seniors to maintain their independence and perform daily activities with ease. Seniors who exercise regularly are more likely to stay mobile and self-sufficient for a longer period.

Improving Sleep: Regular physical activity promotes better sleep patterns, helping seniors fall asleep faster and enjoy deeper, more restorative sleep.Adequate sleep is crucial for one's overall health and state of well-being.

Strengthening Immune System: Regular exercise can boost the immune system, making seniors less susceptible to illnesses and infections. It can also speed up the recovery process for seniors who do fall ill.

Enhancing Social Connections: Group exercise classes or activities provide opportunities for social interaction and can help combat feelings of loneliness and isolation. Building friendships and a sense of community can significantly contribute to a senior's emotional well-being.

Increasing Longevity: Studies have shown that regular physical activity is linked to increased lifespan. Seniors who engage in regular exercise tend to live longer, healthier lives compared to those who are sedentary.

Pain Management: Exercise can alleviate chronic pain by strengthening the muscles around affected joints and improving overall flexibility. This can reduce discomfort and enhance the overall quality of life for seniors dealing with pain issues.

In summary, regular exercise is essential for seniors as it not only improves physical health but also has profound positive effects on mental and emotional well-being. It empowers seniors to lead active, fulfilling lives, promoting independence, and enhancing their overall quality of life in the golden years.

Challenges faced by seniors in maintaining fitness levels

Seniors face various challenges when it comes to maintaining their fitness levels. These challenges can be physical, psychological, or environmental in nature. Here are some common challenges faced by seniors in maintaining their fitness levels:

Reduced Muscle Mass and Bone Density: As people age, they naturally lose muscle mass and bone density, making it harder to engage in physical activities and maintain strength.

Joint Problems: Conditions like arthritis can cause pain and stiffness in the joints, making movements uncomfortable and discouraging seniors from exercising.

Chronic Health Conditions: Seniors often deal with chronic health issues such as diabetes, heart disease, or respiratory problems, which may limit their ability to engage in certain types of exercises.

Balance Issues: Reduced balance and stability increase the risk of falls, making seniors cautious about engaging in physical activities that could potentially lead to injuries.

Fear of Injury: Seniors might fear getting injured during exercise, especially if they have experienced falls or injuries in the past. This fear can deter them from engaging in physical activities.

Lack of Motivation: Loneliness, depression, or lack of social interaction can lead to a lack of motivation to exercise regularly. Social isolation can make it challenging to stay active and engaged.

Financial Constraints: Limited financial resources might restrict access to fitness facilities, classes, or equipment, making it difficult for seniors to participate in organized fitness programs.

Cognitive Decline: Cognitive decline, including conditions like dementia, can make it challenging for seniors to remember exercise routines or follow instructions, hindering their ability to maintain a fitness regimen.

Medications: Some medications can cause fatigue, dizziness, or other side effects that make it difficult for seniors to engage in physical activities comfortably.

Limited Mobility: Mobility issues, such as difficulty walking or using stairs, can severely limit the types of exercises seniors can perform, affecting their overall fitness levels.

Nutritional Challenges: Poor nutrition can impact energy levels and overall health, making it harder for seniors to engage in physical activities effectively.

Vision and Hearing Impairments: Impaired vision or hearing can affect a senior's ability to participate in group fitness classes or outdoor activities, limiting their options for staying active.

Addressing these challenges requires tailored fitness programs, regular medical check-ups, social support, and modifications in exercise routines to accommodate individual needs and abilities. Encouragement from family members, caregivers, and healthcare professionals also plays a vital role in helping seniors overcome these challenges and maintain their fitness levels for a healthier lifestyle.

Purpose of the guide: providing practical and effective workout strategies tailored for seniors

The purpose of the guide, "Providing Practical and Effective Workout Strategies Tailored for Seniors," is to empower older adults with the knowledge and tools necessary to maintain and improve their physical fitness, overall health, and well-being. This comprehensive guide aims to address the specific needs, challenges, and goals of seniors by offering specialized workout strategies designed with their unique requirements in mind. Here are the key objectives and goals of this guide:

Promoting Health and Longevity: The guide aims to promote the overall health and longevity of seniors by encouraging regular physical activity. Engaging in appropriate exercises can help seniors manage chronic conditions, maintain a healthy weight, and reduce the risk of age-related diseases.

Enhancing Mobility and Flexibility: Tailored workout strategies focus on improving mobility and flexibility, helping seniors maintain their independence and perform daily tasks with ease. Enhanced mobility also reduces the risk of falls and injuries.

Increasing Strength and Balance: The guide provides exercises that target strength and balance, addressing common issues like muscle weakness and balance problems. Strengthening these areas can enhance stability, making it easier for seniors to move around safely.

Managing Chronic Conditions: Seniors often deal with various chronic conditions such as arthritis, diabetes, and heart disease. The guide offers exercises and fitness routines that can help manage these conditions, alleviate symptoms, and improve overall quality of life.

Boosting Mental Well-being: Regular physical activity has proven benefits for mental health. The guide includes exercises that promote the release of endorphins, reducing stress, anxiety, and depression among seniors. It also emphasizes the importance of mindfulness and relaxation techniques.

Providing Practical and Feasible Workouts: Recognizing the limitations and challenges faced by seniors, the guide offers practical, realistic, and achievable workout routines. These exercises can be performed at home or in a senior-friendly fitness facility, using minimal equipment and focusing on body weight exercises, resistance bands, and light dumbbells.

Ensuring Safety: Safety is a top priority. The guide includes detailed instructions on proper form and technique, ensuring that seniors perform exercises correctly to prevent injuries. It also provides guidelines on how to start gradually and progress safely to more challenging workouts.

Encouraging Social Engagement: The guide promotes social engagement by encouraging seniors to participate in group exercises, classes, or activities. Social interaction boosts motivation, provides a support network, and enhances the overall experience of staying active.

Empowering Self-Care: By providing seniors with tailored workout strategies, the guide empowers them to take control of their own health and fitness. It encourages a proactive approach to self-care, enabling seniors to make informed decisions about their well-being.

Improving Quality of Life: Ultimately, the guide's purpose is to enhance the quality of life for seniors. By promoting physical activity, mental well-being, and social engagement, it enables seniors to lead fulfilling lives, maintain their independence, and enjoy their golden years to the fullest.

CHAPTER 1

Understanding Senior Fitness Needs

Understanding senior fitness needs is essential for developing effective and tailored exercise programs that cater to the unique requirements of older adults. Here's an overview of key considerations when it comes to senior fitness needs:

Individual Variability: Seniors have diverse fitness levels, health conditions, and physical abilities. Understanding these individual differences is crucial to designing personalized fitness plans that address specific needs and limitations.

Health Conditions: Many seniors manage chronic health conditions such as arthritis, diabetes, osteoporosis, and heart disease. Fitness programs should be adapted to accommodate these conditions, ensuring exercises are safe and beneficial.

Mobility and Flexibility: Aging often leads to reduced joint flexibility and mobility. Senior fitness programs should incorporate exercises that enhance range of motion, joint flexibility, and overall mobility, promoting independence in daily activities.

Strength and Balance: Muscle mass and bone density tend to decrease with age, affecting strength and balance. Resistance training exercises can help improve muscular strength, while balance exercises reduce the risk of falls, a common concern among seniors.

Cognitive Health: Exercise has been linked to improved cognitive function and reduced risk of dementia in older adults. Senior fitness programs should include activities that challenge the brain, such as coordination exercises and memory games, to support cognitive well-being.

Cardiovascular Health: Regular aerobic exercises, tailored to seniors' fitness levels, help improve cardiovascular health, stamina, and endurance. Activities like walking, swimming, or cycling can be adapted to accommodate different fitness levels.

Bone Health: Osteoporosis, a condition characterized by weakened bones, is prevalent among seniors, especially women. Weight-bearing exercises and resistance training can aid in maintaining bone density and reducing the risk of fractures.

Pain Management: Seniors often experience pain, particularly in joints and muscles. Fitness programs should focus on gentle exercises, stretching, and low-impact activities to manage pain effectively without exacerbating existing conditions.

Social Engagement: Loneliness and social isolation can negatively impact seniors' mental and emotional well-being. Group fitness classes or activities encourage social interaction, fostering a sense of community and motivation to stay active.

<u>Safety Concerns:</u> Seniors may have concerns about safety during physical activities. It is important to create an environment where they feel secure, providing proper guidance on techniques and equipment usage to prevent injuries.

<u>Regular Monitoring:</u> Regular assessments and monitoring of seniors' progress are vital. Fitness professionals should track their clients' achievements, adjust workout routines based on progress, and be vigilant about any signs of discomfort or fatigue.

<u>Motivation and Support:</u> Seniors often require motivation and emotional support to adhere to fitness routines. Encouragement from trainers, caregivers, or peers can significantly impact their commitment to regular exercise.

By understanding these specific needs, fitness professionals and caregivers can design programs that cater to the holistic well-being of seniors, promoting their physical, mental, and emotional health, and ensuring a higher quality of life as they age.

<u>**Physiological changes associated with aging**</u>

Aging is a natural and inevitable process that brings about various physiological changes in the human body. These changes occur at different rates for different individuals but generally follow similar patterns. Here are some of the key physiological changes associated with aging:

Muscle Mass and Strength: As people age, there is a gradual loss of muscle mass and a decline in muscle strength. This process, known as sarcopenia, can result in reduced mobility and increased frailty.

Bone Density: Bone density tends to decrease with age, leading to a higher risk of osteoporosis and fractures. This decrease in bone density is more common in women after menopause due to hormonal changes.

Metabolism: Metabolic rate typically slows down with age. This indicates that the body expends fewer calories while at rest, posing a greater challenge for weight management.Changes in metabolism can also affect energy levels and overall vitality.

Cardiovascular System: Aging can lead to stiffening of blood vessels, increased blood pressure, and changes in cholesterol levels. These factors contribute to a higher risk of heart disease and other cardiovascular conditions.

Respiratory System: Lung elasticity decreases, leading to reduced lung capacity and a decreased ability to oxygenate the blood. This can result in reduced stamina and endurance.

Vision: Aging often leads to changes in vision, including difficulty focusing on close objects (presbyopia), reduced peripheral vision, and an increased risk of conditions such as cataracts and macular degeneration.

Hearing: Hearing loss is a common age-related issue. It often starts with difficulty hearing high-pitched sounds and can progress to more significant hearing loss over time.

Digestive System: The digestive system may become less efficient, leading to issues such as constipation and decreased absorption of certain nutrients. Changes in taste and smell can also affect appetite and nutrition.

Hormonal Changes: Women experience menopause, leading to a decline in estrogen levels, while men may experience a gradual decline in testosterone levels. These hormonal changes can have various effects on the body, including changes in bone density and muscle mass.

Nervous System: Aging can affect the nervous system, leading to a decrease in the number of nerve cells and a slower transmission of nerve impulses. This can result in a decline in reaction time and coordination.

Immune System: The immune system becomes less efficient with age, leading to a higher susceptibility to infections and a decreased ability to fight off illnesses.

Cognitive Function: While aging does not necessarily lead to dementia, cognitive functions such as memory, processing speed, and multitasking abilities may decline gradually. However, a healthy lifestyle, including mental stimulation and social engagement, can help preserve cognitive function.

It's important to note that while these physiological changes are a natural part of the aging process, a healthy lifestyle, including regular exercise, balanced nutrition, and regular medical check-ups, can significantly impact the rate and extent of these changes, allowing individuals to lead fulfilling and active lives as they age.

Common health concerns and their impact on exercise

Common health concerns can significantly impact the ability of seniors to engage in regular exercise. These health issues often pose challenges and require careful consideration when designing fitness programs for older adults. Here are some common health concerns and their impact on exercise for seniors:

Arthritis: Arthritis causes joint pain and stiffness, making high-impact exercises uncomfortable. Seniors with arthritis may benefit from low-impact activities like swimming or stationary biking, which are gentle on the joints.

Cardiovascular Issues: Conditions such as high blood pressure, heart disease, or a history of stroke require careful monitoring during exercise. Seniors should engage in moderate-intensity aerobic activities, with close attention to their heart rate and blood pressure.

Osteoporosis: Reduced bone strength caused by osteoporosis raises the likelihood of fractures. Engaging in weight-bearing exercises and resistance training can enhance bone density, but it's crucial to steer clear of high-impact activities to prevent injuries.

Diabetes: Older adults dealing with diabetes must regulate their blood sugar levels while exercising. Consistent physical activity can enhance insulin sensitivity. Nevertheless, it's important for them to keep track of their blood glucose levels and modify their workout regimen as needed.

Chronic Respiratory Conditions: Seniors with conditions like chronic obstructive pulmonary disease (COPD) may experience shortness of breath. Low-intensity aerobic exercises and breathing exercises can help improve lung function and endurance.

<u>Neurological Disorders</u>: Conditions like Parkinson's disease or multiple sclerosis can affect mobility and coordination. Exercise programs should focus on improving balance, strength, and flexibility to enhance overall motor skills.

<u>Cognitive Impairment:</u> Seniors with cognitive impairments, such as dementia, may require exercises that are easy to follow and provide mental stimulation. Simple activities like seated exercises, walking, or dancing can be beneficial.

<u>Depression and Anxiety:</u> Mental health concerns can affect motivation and participation in physical activities. Regular exercise has proven benefits for mental health, reducing symptoms of depression and anxiety. Group exercises or activities that encourage social interaction can be particularly beneficial.

Obesity: Obesity can exacerbate joint problems and cardiovascular issues. Seniors with obesity may start with low-impact exercises and gradually increase intensity as their fitness improves. A combination of aerobic and resistance training can aid in weight management.

Vision and Hearing Impairments: Seniors with vision or hearing impairments may need exercises that do not rely heavily on visual or auditory cues. Instructors should provide clear, simple instructions and consider adaptations for those with sensory impairments.

Medications: Certain medications can affect energy levels, balance, or hydration. Seniors should be aware of the side effects of their medications and adapt their exercise routines accordingly, especially if they experience dizziness or fatigue.

Tailoring exercise programs to address these specific health concerns ensures that seniors can reap the benefits of physical activity while minimizing the risk of exacerbating their existing conditions. Consulting healthcare professionals or certified trainers experienced in senior fitness is crucial to developing safe and effective exercise plans for older adults.

Benefits of age-appropriate workouts, including improved strength, balance, and flexibility

Engaging in age-appropriate workouts offers a wide range of benefits for seniors, focusing on improving strength, balance, and flexibility. Here are some key advantages:

Improved Strength:

Age-appropriate exercises help seniors build and maintain muscle strength. This is crucial for performing daily activities, such as carrying groceries or getting up from a chair, without experiencing fatigue or strain.

Stronger muscles also support joint health, reducing the risk of arthritis and other joint-related issues.

Enhanced Balance:

Balance exercises are integral for seniors as they age because they help prevent falls, which can have severe consequences for older adults.

Improving balance through specific workouts reduces the risk of accidents, enhancing overall stability and confidence in movement.

Increased Flexibility:

Stretching exercises incorporated into workouts can improve flexibility and range of motion in joints.

Enhanced flexibility allows seniors to maintain better posture, move more freely, and perform various activities with greater ease.

Reduced Risk of Injury:

Age-appropriate workouts are designed to be gentle on joints and tailored to individual fitness levels, reducing the risk of injuries commonly associated with high-impact exercises.

By focusing on low-impact, controlled movements, seniors can exercise safely and effectively, minimizing the chance of strains or sprains.

Enhanced Joint Health:

Regular, gentle exercises help lubricate the joints, promoting better mobility and reducing stiffness.

Strengthening the muscles around joints provides additional support, alleviating pressure on the joints and reducing the risk of conditions like osteoarthritis.

Improved Mental Well-being:

Engaging in physical activity has been proven to trigger the release of endorphins, which are the body's natural mood-enhancing chemicals.Regular physical activity can help seniors combat symptoms of depression and anxiety.

Participating in age-appropriate workouts in a social setting, such as group classes, can also provide a sense of community and support, reducing feelings of isolation.

<u>Better Cardiovascular Health:</u>

Cardiovascular exercises, adapted to seniors' needs, contribute to a healthy heart and improved circulation.

A strong cardiovascular system ensures that the body's organs, muscles, and tissues receive an adequate supply of oxygen and nutrients, supporting overall vitality.

<u>Enhanced Quality of Life:</u>

By improving strength, balance, and flexibility, seniors can maintain their independence and continue to enjoy their favorite activities and hobbies.

A higher level of physical fitness enables seniors to engage in daily tasks without assistance, leading to an improved quality of life and a sense of accomplishment.

In summary, age-appropriate workouts play a crucial role in enhancing the overall well-being of seniors, offering physical, mental, and emotional benefits that contribute to a healthier and more active lifestyle in the golden years.

CHAPTER 2

Preparing for Safe Exercise

As we grow older, it becomes more crucial to engage in regular physical activity to preserve good health and overall wellness.Regular exercise can improve strength, flexibility, balance, and cardiovascular health in seniors. However, safety should always be a top priority to prevent injuries and promote a positive exercise experience. This guide provides valuable information on preparing for safe exercise tailored specifically for seniors.

Section 1: Consultation with Healthcare Professionals

1.1 Schedule a Check-up:

Visit your healthcare provider for a thorough health assessment before starting any exercise program.

Discuss any existing medical conditions, medications, or concerns to receive personalized exercise recommendations.

1.2 Physical Therapy Consultation:

Consider consulting a physical therapist to assess your mobility, strength, and balance.

They can design a customized exercise plan addressing specific needs and limitations.

Section 2: Choosing the Right Exercises

2.1 Low-Impact Activities:

Opt for low-impact exercises like walking, swimming, or cycling to reduce stress on joints and minimize the risk of injury.

Incorporate chair exercises and resistance band workouts for added support.

2.2 Balance and Flexibility Exercises:

Practice balance exercises to improve stability and prevent falls.

Include stretching routines to enhance flexibility and maintain joint mobility.

Section 3:Creating a Safe Exercise Environment

3.1 Proper Warm-up and Cool-down:

Begin each session with a mild warm-up to ready your muscles and joints for physical activity.Conclude each session with a cool-down period and gentle stretches to relax the body.

3.2 Safe Equipment Use:

Use sturdy and well-maintained footwear to provide proper support and reduce the risk of slipping.
Ensure exercise equipment is stable and adjusted to your body size to prevent accidents.

Section 4: Listening to Your Body

4.1 Recognizing Pain and Discomfort:

Learn to differentiate between muscle fatigue and pain. Cease physical activity if you feel sharp or continuous pain. Be attentive to your body's cues and modify your workout routine accordingly.

4.2 Rest and Recovery:

Allow ample time for rest and recovery between exercise sessions to prevent overexertion and promote muscle recovery.
Adequate sleep and hydration are crucial for overall well-being and exercise performance.

By following these guidelines and prioritizing safety, seniors can enjoy the numerous benefits of regular exercise. Always consult healthcare professionals, choose appropriate exercises, create a safe environment, and listen to your body's cues. With proper preparation and caution, seniors can maintain an active and healthy lifestyle for years to come.

Consultation with healthcare professionals before starting any workout routine

Prior to embarking on a workout routine, it is essential for seniors to consult healthcare professionals to ensure their safety and well-being during physical activity. This consultation provides personalized guidance, taking into account individual health conditions, limitations, and specific needs. Here's why consulting healthcare professionals is paramount for seniors beginning a workout regimen.

Comprehensive Health Assessment:

Healthcare professionals conduct thorough evaluations to assess existing medical conditions, medications, and overall health status.

They consider factors such as cardiovascular health, joint mobility, and muscular strength to tailor exercise recommendations accordingly.

Personalized Exercise Recommendations:

Based on the health assessment, professionals provide customized exercise plans designed to address specific concerns and limitations.

These tailored recommendations ensure that seniors engage in exercises that are safe, effective, and beneficial for their individual health goals.

Management of Chronic Conditions:

Healthcare professionals can offer guidance on managing chronic conditions such as arthritis, diabetes, or heart disease through suitable exercises.

They can recommend exercises that help improve symptoms and enhance overall well-being, while minimizing the risk of exacerbating health issues.

Injury Prevention:

Professionals can identify potential risks and recommend exercises that reduce the risk of injury, especially for seniors with joint problems or previous injuries.

Proper guidance helps seniors perform exercises with correct form, reducing the likelihood of strains or sprains.

Regular Monitoring and Progression:

Healthcare professionals can monitor progress over time and adjust the exercise routine accordingly.

Regular follow-ups ensure that the workout routine remains effective, safe, and aligned with the senior's changing health needs.

Consulting healthcare professionals before starting a workout routine is a fundamental step in promoting the well-being of seniors. Their expertise ensures that seniors engage in exercises suitable for their individual health conditions, enhancing the benefits of physical activity while minimizing risks. By seeking professional guidance, seniors can enjoy a safe and tailored approach to staying active, leading to improved overall health and quality of life.

Importance of warm-up and cool-down exercises

Warm-up and cool-down exercises are integral components of any fitness routine, especially for seniors. These preparatory and concluding exercises play a vital role in ensuring the safety, effectiveness, and overall well-being of older adults during physical activities. This article explores the importance of warm-up and cool-down exercises for seniors and their impact on promoting a healthy and active lifestyle.

Preventing Injury:

Warm-up: Gentle warm-up exercises increase blood flow to muscles, making them more pliable and less prone to injury. This is particularly important for seniors, as it helps prepare their bodies for more intense physical activity, reducing the risk of strains and sprains.

Cool-down: Cooling down gradually decreases heart rate and helps prevent abrupt stops in physical activity, reducing the risk of dizziness and muscle cramps.

Improved Flexibility and Mobility:

Warm-up: Dynamic stretching during warm-up routines enhances flexibility and joint mobility, allowing seniors to move more freely during their workout sessions.

Cool-down: Incorporating static stretches during the cool-down phase helps maintain and improve flexibility over time, contributing to better overall mobility in daily activities.

Enhanced Performance:

Warm-up: A proper warm-up primes the cardiovascular system, enabling the heart to pump more blood and oxygen to muscles. This increased circulation enhances endurance and performance during exercises.

Cool-down: Gradual reduction in intensity helps prevent rapid fatigue, allowing seniors to sustain their workout efforts and achieve their fitness goals more effectively.

Muscle Recovery and Relaxation:

Warm-up: Engaging in light aerobic activities warms up the muscles, making them more receptive to stretching and reducing the risk of muscle strain.

Cool-down: Gentle exercises during the cool-down period promote relaxation and alleviate muscle tension. This relaxation aids in quicker recovery and reduces post-workout soreness.

Mental Preparation and Stress Reduction:

Warm-up: The warm-up phase offers an opportunity for seniors to mentally prepare for their workout, focusing on their goals and increasing motivation.

Cool-down: Cooling down with calming exercises and deep breathing techniques helps seniors relax, reducing stress and promoting a sense of well-being.

Warm-up and cool-down exercises are essential elements of a safe and effective workout routine for seniors. By incorporating these practices into their physical activities, older adults can minimize the risk of injuries, improve flexibility, enhance performance, aid muscle recovery, and reduce stress. Emphasizing the importance of warm-up and cool-down exercises empowers seniors to maintain an active and healthy lifestyle, ensuring their overall well-being in the long run.

Choosing suitable workout attire and footwear for safety and comfort

Choosing appropriate workout attire and footwear is crucial for ensuring the safety and comfort of seniors during physical activities. Proper clothing and shoes not only enhance mobility but also reduce the risk of injuries, allowing older adults to engage in exercise routines comfortably. This guide provides essential tips on selecting suitable workout attire and footwear tailored to the specific needs of seniors.

Comfortable and Breathable Fabrics:

Seniors should opt for workout clothes made from breathable and moisture-wicking fabrics such as cotton blends or specialized performance materials. Loose-fitting attire allows for easy movement and promotes air circulation, preventing overheating during exercises.

Appropriate Layers:

Dressing in layers enables seniors to adjust their clothing according to the temperature and intensity of their workout.

Lightweight layers can be added or removed as needed, ensuring comfort throughout the exercise session.

Supportive Sports Bras:

For women, choosing a supportive sports bra is essential to reduce breast movement and discomfort during physical activities.

Proper support minimizes strain on the back and chest muscles, enhancing overall comfort during workouts.

Proper Footwear:

Seniors should wear athletic shoes specifically designed for their chosen activity, whether it's walking, jogging, or strength training.

Shoes should provide adequate arch support, cushioning, and stability to reduce the risk of falls and foot-related injuries.

Correct Socks:

Seniors should wear moisture-wicking socks that help prevent blisters and keep the feet dry.

Avoiding cotton socks, which retain moisture, can reduce the likelihood of friction and discomfort.

Grippy Soles:

Pay attention to the sole grip of athletic shoes, especially for activities like walking or aerobics.

Shoes with non-slip, rubber soles provide stability and reduce the risk of slipping, ensuring safe movement during exercises.

Proper Shoe Fit:

Seniors should have their feet measured regularly to ensure they wear shoes of the correct size.

Shoes should have a thumb's width of space between the longest toe and the shoe tip, allowing for natural movement and preventing discomfort.

Selecting suitable workout attire and footwear is essential for the safety and comfort of seniors during physical activities. By choosing breathable fabrics, appropriate layers, supportive sports bras, and well-fitted, grippy footwear, older adults can enjoy their exercises with reduced risk of injury and enhanced comfort. Prioritizing the right clothing and shoes empowers seniors to engage in regular physical activity, promoting their overall health and well-being.

CHAPTER 3

Low-Impact and Senior-Friendly Exercises

For seniors, engaging in low-impact and senior-friendly exercises is a fantastic way to promote physical health, improve flexibility, and boost overall well-being. These exercises are gentle on the joints and muscles, making them ideal for older adults who may have mobility limitations. In this guide, we explore a variety of low-impact activities tailored specifically to seniors, ensuring they can stay active and healthy at any age.

Walking:

Walking is a simple and effective low-impact exercise that can be adapted to various fitness levels.

Seniors can enjoy strolls in the neighborhood, local parks, or indoor malls to improve cardiovascular health and maintain joint mobility.

Swimming and Water Aerobics:

Water-based exercises, such as swimming and water aerobics, provide resistance without putting stress on the joints.

Water activities enhance muscle strength, cardiovascular endurance, and flexibility while reducing the risk of impact-related injuries.

Chair Exercises:

Chair exercises are excellent for seniors with limited mobility or balance issues.
Seated marches, seated leg lifts, and seated torso twists can be done safely, promoting strength and flexibility.

Tai Chi:

Tai Chi is a low-impact exercise that combines gentle movements and deep breathing.
This ancient Chinese practice improves balance, flexibility, and mental well-being, making it ideal for seniors seeking mind-body harmony.

<u>Yoga:</u>

Yoga offers various poses and stretches that can be modified to accommodate different abilities.

Practicing yoga enhances balance, flexibility, and strength, while also promoting relaxation and stress reduction.

<u>Cycling:</u>

Stationary bikes or recumbent bikes provide a low-impact cardiovascular workout.

Cycling strengthens leg muscles and improves endurance without putting pressure on the joints, making it suitable for seniors.

<u>Resistance Band Exercises:</u>

Resistance bands offer gentle resistance for strength training without heavy weights.

Seniors can perform exercises like bicep curls, leg lifts, and shoulder presses to build muscle and improve overall body tone.

Low-impact and senior-friendly exercises empower older adults to maintain an active lifestyle while minimizing the risk of injuries. By incorporating activities like walking, swimming, chair exercises, Tai Chi, yoga, cycling, and resistance band workouts into their routine, seniors can enhance their physical fitness, flexibility, and mental well-being. These exercises not only promote overall health but also contribute to a sense of accomplishment and improved quality of life in their golden years.

Gentle cardiovascular exercises (e.g., walking, swimming)

Engaging in gentle cardiovascular exercises is a fantastic way for seniors to maintain heart health, improve circulation, and boost overall well-being. Activities like walking and swimming provide an effective cardiovascular workout without putting excessive strain on joints and muscles. This guide explores the benefits of gentle cardiovascular exercises for seniors and provides practical tips on incorporating activities such as walking and swimming into their routine.

Walking:

Walking is a low-impact exercise that can be easily adapted to various fitness levels.

Seniors can start with short, leisurely walks and gradually increase the duration and intensity as their stamina improves.

Walking strengthens the heart, improves lung capacity, and supports joint flexibility, making it an ideal cardiovascular activity for older adults.

Swimming:

Swimming is a highly effective and gentle cardiovascular exercise that provides a full-body workout.

The buoyancy of water reduces impact on joints, making it suitable for seniors with arthritis or joint pain.

Seniors can enjoy different strokes like freestyle, breaststroke, or backstroke, tailoring their swimming routine to their comfort level and preferences.

Water Aerobics:

Water aerobics combines cardiovascular exercises with resistance training in a low-impact aquatic environment.

Seniors can participate in water aerobics classes specifically designed for their age group, improving cardiovascular health while working on muscle tone and flexibility.

Dance Aerobics:

Dance aerobics classes designed for seniors incorporate rhythmic movements to lively music, making exercise enjoyable and engaging.

These classes enhance cardiovascular endurance, balance, and coordination while providing a social and fun atmosphere for seniors.

Stationary Cycling:

Stationary bikes offer a low-impact way to engage in cardiovascular exercises.

Seniors can cycle at a comfortable pace, adjusting the resistance level as needed, to improve heart health and leg strength without stressing the joints.

<u>Elliptical Trainer:</u>

Elliptical trainers provide a smooth, gliding motion that mimics walking or running without the impact on joints.

Seniors can use elliptical trainers to enhance cardiovascular endurance and burn calories in a gentle and controlled manner.

Gentle cardiovascular exercises such as walking, swimming, water aerobics, dance aerobics, stationary cycling, and elliptical training offer numerous health benefits for seniors. These activities improve heart health, increase lung capacity, and support overall fitness while minimizing the risk of injury. Encouraging seniors to participate in these gentle exercises not only promotes physical well-being but also enhances their mental and emotional health, fostering a sense of accomplishment and vitality in their daily lives.

Strength training with light weights or resistance bands

Strength training plays a pivotal role in maintaining muscle mass, bone density, and overall functional independence as we age. For seniors, incorporating light weights and resistance bands into their exercise routine offers a safe and effective way to build strength and enhance physical well-being. This guide explores the benefits and techniques of strength training with light weights and resistance bands specifically tailored for seniors.

Benefits of Strength Training for Seniors:

Improved Muscle Strength: Enhances muscle tone and power, making daily tasks easier.

Enhanced Bone Density: Strength training helps maintain bone mass, reducing the risk of osteoporosis.

Joint Health: Strengthens the muscles around joints, providing support and reducing the risk of injuries.

Improved Balance: Builds core muscles, enhancing stability and reducing the risk of falls.

Boosted Metabolism: Increases muscle mass, promoting a higher resting metabolic rate, aiding in weight management.

Getting Started:

Consult a Professional: Seniors should consult a fitness trainer or physical therapist to design a personalized strength training program based on individual fitness levels and health conditions.

Warm-up: Begin each session with a gentle warm-up, involving light cardio activities and dynamic stretches to prepare the muscles for exercise.

Light Weights:

Choosing the Right Weight: Opt for light dumbbells or resistance bands with adjustable tension.

Proper Form: Focus on proper form and controlled movements to target specific muscle groupsBegin by performing each exercise for 10-15 repetitions in **1-2 sets.Exercises:** Include exercises like bicep curls, shoulder presses, tricep extensions, and leg lifts using light weights to target different muscle groups.

Resistance Bands:

Variable Resistance: Resistance bands offer adjustable tension levels, allowing seniors to customize the intensity of their workouts.

Versatility: Bands can be used for various exercises, including chest presses, rows, squats, and leg lifts, providing a full-body workout.
Stability: Bands promote stability as they engage stabilizing muscles, improving overall balance and coordination.

<u>Cool-down and Stretching:</u>

Cool-down: After the session, engage in gentle aerobic activities followed by static stretches to cool down the body and improve flexibility.

Stretching: Perform stretches targeting major muscle groups to enhance flexibility and prevent muscle stiffness.

Strength training with light weights and resistance bands offers seniors a safe and effective way to maintain muscle strength, improve balance, and support overall physical health. By incorporating these exercises into their routine, seniors can enjoy the benefits of enhanced strength and flexibility, promoting a healthier and more active lifestyle as they age. It is essential to follow proper techniques, consult professionals, and listen to the body to ensure a safe and rewarding strength training experience.

<u>Balance and flexibility exercises (e.g., yoga, tai chi)</u>

Maintaining balance and flexibility is crucial for seniors to prevent falls, improve mobility, and enhance overall well-being. Engaging in exercises like yoga and Tai Chi offers gentle yet effective ways for older adults to boost balance, flexibility, and coordination. This guide explores these senior-friendly exercises, emphasizing their benefits and techniques tailored to enhance balance and flexibility in older individuals.

<u>Yoga for Seniors:</u>

Gentle Poses: Yoga poses can be modified to suit seniors, focusing on gentle stretches and balance-enhancing postures.

<u>Breathing Exercises:</u> Incorporate breathing exercises (pranayama) to promote relaxation, reduce stress, and improve lung capacity.

Chair Yoga: Chair yoga adapts traditional poses, allowing seniors to practice yoga while seated, providing support and stability.

Balance Poses: Include balance poses like Tree Pose and Warrior III, enhancing stability and concentration while strengthening leg muscles.

Tai Chi for Seniors:

Slow, Flowing Movements: Tai Chi involves slow, continuous movements that improve balance, coordination, and joint flexibility.

Focus on Breathing: Emphasize deep breathing techniques, synchronizing breath with movement to enhance relaxation and concentration.

Weight Shifting Exercises: Practice weight shifting exercises to improve stability, shifting body weight from one leg to another in controlled motions.

Mind-Body Connection: Tai Chi fosters a strong mind-body connection, promoting mental clarity and reducing anxiety.

Benefits of Balance and Flexibility Exercises:

Improved Stability: Enhances balance, reducing the risk of falls and injuries, especially in seniors.

Enhanced Flexibility: Increases joint range of motion, making daily activities easier and more comfortable.

Better Posture: Promotes proper body alignment, reducing strain on muscles and joints.

Pain Relief: Alleviates joint and muscle pain by promoting relaxation and reducing muscle tension.

Mental Well-being: Enhances mental focus, reduces stress, and promotes a sense of calm and well-being.

Safety Precautions:

Start Slow: Begin with basic poses and gradually progress to more advanced movements as confidence and strength improve.

Use Props: Utilize props like yoga blocks or chairs for support and balance during exercises.

Consult Professionals: Seniors with existing health conditions or concerns should consult healthcare professionals or experienced instructors for guidance.

Balance and flexibility exercises, such as yoga and Tai Chi, offer seniors the opportunity to enhance their physical and mental well-being in a gentle and enjoyable manner. By incorporating these practices into their routine, older adults can experience improved stability, flexibility, and overall vitality, enabling them to lead a more active and fulfilling lifestyle as they age. It is essential to practice these exercises mindfully, focusing on proper techniques and individual comfort, to reap the maximum benefits and promote long-term health and wellness.

Chair exercises and seated workouts for seniors with limited mobility

For seniors with limited mobility, chair exercises and seated workouts offer a convenient and effective way to stay active, improve strength, and enhance overall well-being. These exercises, designed to be performed while sitting, provide a safe and supportive environment for older adults, allowing them to maintain their fitness levels and mobility. In this guide, we explore a variety of chair exercises and seated workouts tailored specifically for seniors with limited mobility.

Seated Marches:

Technique: Sit upright and lift one knee toward your chest, then lower it and lift the other knee. Repeat this motion, as if you're marching in place.

Benefits: Strengthens leg muscles and improves circulation, promoting cardiovascular health.

Seated Leg Lifts:

Technique: Sit with your back straight, lift one leg straight out in front of you, hold briefly, and lower it. Alternate between legs.

Benefits: Targets thigh muscles and enhances hip flexibility, aiding in mobility.

Seated Torso Twists:

Technique: Sit tall and twist your torso gently to one side, hold for a few seconds, return to the center, and twist to the other side.

Benefits: Improves spinal flexibility and strengthens core muscles, enhancing balance.

Chair Squats:

Technique: Stand in front of a sturdy chair, lower your body as if you're about to sit, then rise back up without fully sitting down.

Benefits: Strengthens leg muscles, especially quadriceps and glutes, while providing support for balance.

Seated Rowing:

Technique: Sit comfortably with your arms extended in front of you, as if holding an oar. Pull your hands towards your chest, engaging your back muscles, and then extend your arms forward again.

Benefits: Targets upper back muscles, enhancing posture and reducing back pain.

<u>Seated Shoulder Press</u>:

Technique: Hold a light weight (or a water bottle) in each hand at shoulder height. Push the weights upward until your arms are fully extended, then lower them back down.

Benefits: Strengthens shoulder muscles and improves upper body mobility.

<u>Seated Stretching Routine:</u>

Technique: Perform gentle stretches for various muscle groups, including neck, shoulders, arms, and legs, to enhance flexibility and relieve muscle tension.

Benefits: Improves overall flexibility, reduces stiffness, and enhances range of motion.

Chair exercises and seated workouts offer a valuable fitness solution for seniors with limited mobility, allowing them to maintain their physical health and mobility in a safe and controlled manner. By incorporating these exercises into their routine, older adults can experience improved strength, flexibility, and overall well-being, fostering a sense of independence and vitality. It is essential to perform these exercises mindfully, focusing on proper form and individual comfort, to maximize the benefits and support long-term health and fitness.

CHAPTER 4

Designing Personalized Workout Plans

Designing a personalized workout plan is essential for seniors to maintain their health, fitness, and overall well-being as they age. A customized approach takes into account individual needs, preferences, and physical limitations, ensuring that the workout routine is safe, enjoyable, and effective. This guide explores the key components of designing personalized workout plans specifically tailored for seniors, promoting a healthier and more active lifestyle in their golden years.

Health Assessment:

Consultation with Professionals: Seniors should begin by consulting healthcare providers, fitness trainers, or physical therapists to assess their current health status and identify any underlying medical conditions or physical limitations.

Individual Health Goals: Determine specific fitness goals, whether it's improving cardiovascular health, building strength, enhancing balance, or managing weight. Tailor the workout plan based on these goals.

Choosing Appropriate Exercises:

Low-Impact Activities: Opt for exercises that are gentle on joints, such as walking, swimming, cycling, and chair exercises, to minimize the risk of injuries.

Strength Training: Incorporate light weights, resistance bands, or bodyweight exercises to maintain muscle mass and improve overall strength.

Balance and Flexibility Training: Include activities like yoga, Tai Chi, or stretching exercises to enhance balance, flexibility, and coordination.

Customizing Intensity and Duration:

Individual Fitness Level: Customize the intensity of exercises based on the senior's fitness level, gradually increasing it as their strength and endurance improve.

Duration and Frequency: Determine the appropriate duration and frequency of workouts, considering factors such as age, fitness level, and any existing health conditions. Start with shorter sessions and gradually extend the duration as the senior becomes more comfortable.

Incorporating Variety and Enjoyment:

Variety in Exercises: Keep the workout routine engaging by incorporating a variety of exercises and activities. This prevents boredom and ensures a well-rounded fitness program.

Social Activities: Encourage participation in group classes or activities to promote social interaction, motivation, and enjoyment in the workout routine.

Safety Precautions:

Proper Form: Emphasize the importance of correct form and technique to prevent injuries. Think about enlisting the help of a trainer for initial assistance.Warm-up and Cool-down: Include appropriate warm-up and cool-down exercises in every session to prepare the body for exercise and aid in recovery.

Listening to the Body: Encourage seniors to listen to their bodies and adjust the workout intensity or duration as needed. It's crucial to avoid overexertion and respect their physical limitations. Regular Monitoring and Adjustments:

Progress Tracking: Regularly monitor progress by keeping track of fitness achievements and making adjustments to the workout plan as necessary.

Flexibility in Approach: Be adaptable and open to modifying the workout plan based on the senior's evolving needs.

Designing a personalized workout plan for seniors is an investment in their health and quality of life. By considering individual health assessments, appropriate exercises, customized intensity, variety, safety precautions, and regular monitoring, seniors can engage in a fitness routine that is enjoyable, effective, and tailored to their unique requirements. A personalized approach ensures that seniors can maintain their physical fitness, independence, and overall well-being, empowering them to lead an active and fulfilling life in their later years.

Assessing individual fitness levels and setting realistic goals

Assessing the fitness levels of seniors and establishing realistic goals is fundamental to creating an effective and safe exercise plan tailored to their unique needs. By understanding their current capabilities and setting achievable objectives, seniors can engage in physical activities that promote overall health and well-being. This guide explores the importance of assessing individual fitness levels and provides insights on setting realistic and attainable goals for seniors.

<u>Comprehensive Fitness Assessment:</u>

Consultation with Professionals: Seniors should consult healthcare providers, fitness trainers, or physical therapists for a comprehensive fitness assessment. This assessment should include evaluating cardiovascular health, strength, flexibility, balance, and any existing health conditions or limitations.

Functional Fitness Tests: Conduct functional assessments, such as timed walks, chair stands, and balance tests, to gauge mobility and functional abilities in real-life situations.

<u>Understanding Limitations and Preferences:</u>

Health Concerns: Take into account any medical conditions, joint problems, or chronic issues that might affect the choice of exercises and intensity levels.

Personal Preferences: Understand the senior's interests and preferences regarding physical activities. Tailoring the workout routine to their likes enhances motivation and adherence.

<u>Setting Realistic and Achievable Goals:</u>

Specific and Measurable Goals: Establish clear, specific, and measurable objectives, such as walking a certain distance, completing a set of exercises, or improving balance duration.

Realistic Expectations: Ensure goals are realistic and attainable within a reasonable timeframe. Setting achievable milestones boosts confidence and motivation.

Gradual Progression: Plan for gradual progression. Start with manageable goals, then gradually increase intensity, duration, or complexity as the senior's fitness level improves.

<u>Diversifying Fitness Goals:</u>

Cardiovascular Health: Focus on goals related to improving cardiovascular health, such as walking a specific number of steps daily or completing a certain duration of low-impact aerobic exercises.

Strength and Balance: Set goals to enhance strength and balance, incorporating resistance exercises and balance training, aiming to reduce the risk of falls.

Flexibility and Mobility: Include goals to improve flexibility through stretching exercises, enhancing joint mobility and range of motion.

<u>Regular Progress Evaluation:</u>

Tracking Progress: Encourage seniors to keep a fitness journal or use fitness apps to track their progress. Regular monitoring provides motivation and a sense of achievement.

Adjusting Goals: Periodically assess the goals and make necessary adjustments based on the senior's progress and changing fitness levels. Celebrate achievements and set new challenges to maintain motivation.

Assessing individual fitness levels and establishing realistic goals empower seniors to embark on a fitness journey that is tailored to their capabilities and aspirations. By understanding their limitations, preferences, and setting achievable objectives, seniors can engage in exercises that enhance their overall health, boost confidence, and improve their quality of life. Regular evaluation and adjustments to their goals ensure a continuous and rewarding fitness experience, promoting long-term well-being and vitality in their senior years.

Creating customized workout routines based on seniors' abilities and preferences

Designing customized workout routines tailored to seniors' abilities and preferences is essential for promoting engagement, motivation, and overall well-being. By understanding their unique strengths, limitations, and interests, personalized exercise plans can be developed to enhance physical health and provide a positive fitness experience. This guide explores the importance of creating customized workout routines for seniors and provides insights into designing exercises that align with their abilities and preferences.

<u>Assessing Abilities and Health Conditions:</u>

Consultation with Professionals: Seek input from healthcare providers, physiotherapists, or fitness trainers to assess seniors' physical abilities, health conditions, and any limitations.

Functional Assessments: Conduct functional assessments to determine mobility, balance, and strength levels, providing a clear understanding of their capabilities.

Understanding Preferences and Interests:

Personal Interests: Consider seniors' hobbies and interests, incorporating activities they enjoy to increase motivation and participation.

Variety: Offer a variety of exercises, ensuring the routine includes activities they find enjoyable, such as dancing, walking in nature, or participating in group fitness classes.

<u>**Designing Tailored Exercises:**</u>

Low-Impact Cardiovascular Activities: Choose low-impact exercises like walking, swimming, or cycling to enhance cardiovascular health without putting excessive stress on joints.

Strength Training: Incorporate light weights, resistance bands, or bodyweight exercises to maintain muscle mass and improve overall strength.

Balance and Flexibility: Include balance exercises like standing on one leg and flexibility exercises such as yoga stretches to improve stability and joint range of motion.

<u>**Adjusting Intensity and Duration**</u>:

Individualized Intensity: Modify the intensity of exercises based on seniors' fitness levels, gradually increasing intensity as their strength and endurance improve.

Appropriate Duration: Determine the suitable duration for workouts, starting with shorter sessions and gradually extending the duration to avoid fatigue.

Encouraging Social Engagement:

Group Activities: Encourage participation in group exercises or classes to foster social interactions, providing emotional support and motivation.

Buddy System: Suggest working out with friends or family members, creating a supportive environment and promoting consistency in exercise routines.

Regular Monitoring and Feedback:

Progress Tracking: Monitor progress through regular assessments and encourage seniors to keep track of their achievements, celebrating milestones along the way.

open Communication: Maintain open communication to understand their comfort levels and preferences, allowing for adjustments to the routine as needed.

Creating customized workout routines based on seniors' abilities and preferences is key to ensuring their engagement, enjoyment, and adherence to fitness activities. By tailoring exercises to their unique strengths and interests, seniors can experience the physical and mental benefits of regular exercise while enhancing their overall quality of life. Personalized fitness plans provide the foundation for a healthier, happier, and more active lifestyle in their senior years.

Adapting exercises for seniors with specific health conditions or physical limitations

Adapting exercises to accommodate seniors with specific health conditions or physical limitations is essential for ensuring their safety, comfort, and overall well-being during physical activities. Tailoring workout routines to address individual needs allows seniors to enjoy the benefits of exercise while minimizing the risk of exacerbating health conditions or causing injuries. This guide explores the importance of adapting exercises for seniors with various health conditions and provides insights into creating inclusive and customized fitness plans.

<u>Understanding Health Conditions:</u>

Consultation with Healthcare Professionals: Seek guidance from healthcare providers or specialists to understand the senior's specific health condition, its implications, and any exercise-related precautions.

Awareness and Education: Educate fitness instructors and caregivers about the seniors' conditions to ensure exercises are adapted appropriately.

<u>Adapting Cardiovascular Exercises:</u>

Heart Conditions: For seniors with heart conditions, focus on low-impact aerobic exercises like walking or swimming, monitoring heart rate and intensity levels.

Hypertension: Avoid exercises that involve heavy lifting or straining and opt for moderate-intensity activities like cycling or gentle aerobics, emphasizing controlled breathing.

Modifying Strength Training Exercises:

Arthritis: Modify strength exercises to avoid stressing affected joints. Opt for low-impact resistance band exercises targeting muscles around arthritic joints.

Osteoporosis: Incorporate weight-bearing exercises to improve bone density, focusing on bodyweight resistance and gentle strength training with light weights.

Addressing Mobility Challenges:

Limited Mobility: Modify exercises by incorporating seated or chair-based movements, focusing on improving range of motion, flexibility, and muscle strength.

Balance Issues: Introduce balance exercises with support, such as holding onto a chair, to enhance stability and prevent falls. Progress gradually as balance improves.

Adapting Flexibility and Stretching Exercises:

Diabetes: Incorporate gentle stretches to enhance flexibility and improve circulation. Emphasize the importance of foot care and proper footwear for diabetic seniors.

Chronic Pain: Focus on gentle stretching and relaxation techniques, encouraging seniors to listen to their bodies and avoid overstretching or straining affected areas.

Mental Health Considerations:

Depression or Anxiety: Include calming activities like yoga, deep breathing exercises, or meditation to reduce stress and promote mental well-being.

Cognitive Impairment: Incorporate simple, repetitive movements and exercises that engage the senses, providing a sensory-rich experience and enhancing cognitive stimulation.

Regular Monitoring and Feedback:

Communication: Maintain open communication with seniors to understand their comfort levels, any discomfort, or changes in health conditions.

Professional Guidance: Consider enlisting the expertise of fitness trainers experienced in working with seniors and adapting exercises for specific health needs.

Adapting exercises for seniors with specific health conditions or physical limitations is crucial for fostering an inclusive and supportive fitness environment. By tailoring workouts to address individual needs, seniors can experience the physical and mental benefits of exercise safely and comfortably. A collaborative approach involving healthcare professionals, caregivers, and knowledgeable fitness instructors ensures that seniors receive the appropriate exercise modifications, promoting their overall health, confidence, and quality of life.

CHAPTER 5

<u>Motivation and Consistency</u>

Staying motivated and consistent in a workout routine is essential for seniors to maintain good health, strength, and overall well-being. Regular exercise not only enhances physical fitness but also boosts mental health and quality of life. In this guide, we'll explore effective strategies tailored to seniors, ensuring they stay motivated and committed to their workout routines.

1. Prioritize Safety:

Before starting any exercise regimen, consult with your healthcare provider or a fitness professional. They can provide personalized recommendations and ensure your workout plan aligns with your health condition and fitness level. Prioritizing safety sets a strong foundation for a consistent and sustainable workout routine.

2. Choose Enjoyable Activities:

Find physical activities that you genuinely enjoy. Whether it's walking, swimming, gentle yoga, or dance classes, selecting exercises that bring you joy increases your motivation to participate regularly. When you look forward to your workouts, consistency becomes natural.

3. Start Slow and Progress Gradually:
Seniors should start with low-impact exercises and gradually increase intensity. Begin with simple movements to build strength and endurance. Setting achievable milestones allows you to measure progress, boosting your motivation to continue and maintain consistency.

4. Establish a Routine:
Consistency thrives on routine. Set specific days and times for your workouts. Integrating exercise into your daily schedule makes it a habit, ensuring you're more likely to stick with it in the long run.Approach your exercise sessions with the same

level of commitment as you would for essential appointments that are unmissable.

5. Buddy Up:

Working out with a friend or family member can make exercising more enjoyable and increase motivation. Having a workout buddy provides accountability and encouragement, making it easier to stay consistent. You can motivate each other and celebrate your progress together.

6. Track Your Progress:

Maintain a record of your workouts either through a dedicated journal or by utilizing fitness applications to monitor your progress.Documenting your exercises, duration, and any improvements you notice creates a sense of accomplishment. When you see how far you've come, it boosts your motivation to continue and maintain consistency in your workouts.

7. Mix It Up:

Avoid monotony by varying your workouts. Try different types of exercises, such as strength training, flexibility exercises, and balance workouts. Mixing up your routine not only keeps things interesting but also targets different muscle groups, ensuring a well-rounded fitness regimen.

8. Reward Yourself:

Set up a reward system for achieving your fitness goals. Treat yourself with something you enjoy, like a relaxing massage, a new book, or spending time with loved ones. Rewarding your efforts reinforces positive behavior, motivating you to stay consistent with your workouts.

9. Stay Positive and Patient:

Progress might be slow, especially as you age, but staying positive and patient is crucial. Recognize your accomplishments, regardless of their size, and practice self-compassion.A positive mindset and patience help you overcome challenges and maintain motivation, ensuring consistency in your workout routine.

10. Listen to Your Body:

Lastly, pay attention to your body's signals.If you experience pain or discomfort, allow yourself the necessary time to rest and recuperate. Overexertion can result in injuries and loss of motivation, so it's essential to listen to your body and avoid pushing too far. Be mindful of your body's needs and adjust your workout routine accordingly, ensuring a safe and consistent approach to staying fit.

Staying motivated and consistent in workouts for seniors is about finding joy in physical activities, establishing routines, seeking support, tracking progress, and being patient with oneself. By incorporating these strategies into your fitness journey, you can maintain a consistent workout routine that contributes to your overall health, happiness, and vitality. Remember, every step you take toward a healthier you is a significant achievement!

Setting achievable goals and tracking progress

Setting achievable goals and tracking progress are essential components of a successful senior workout routine. Here's how you can approach it:

Setting Achievable Goals:

Be Realistic: Set goals that are attainable considering your current fitness level and health condition. Avoid aiming for drastic changes and focus on gradual improvements.

Specific and Measurable Goals: Define your goals clearly. Instead of a vague goal like "improve fitness," aim for something specific like "walk for 30 minutes without a break" or "perform 10 bodyweight squats."

Short-Term and Long-Term Goals: Break down your fitness journey into short-term goals (achievable within a few weeks or months) and long-term goals (achievable within several months or a year). Short-term goals provide milestones to celebrate, keeping you motivated, while long-term goals provide a sense of direction.

Focus on Different Aspects: Consider goals related to cardiovascular endurance, strength, flexibility, balance, or overall well-being. Diversifying your goals ensures a holistic approach to your fitness routine.

Tracking Progress:

Maintain a Workout Journal: Record your exercises, duration, and any observations after each session. Include details like the number of repetitions, distance covered, or weights used. This journal serves as a reference point to gauge your progress over time.

Use Fitness Apps: Utilize user-friendly fitness applications tailored for seniors. These apps often come with features to log workouts, set reminders, and track progress. They can provide insights into your improvements and help you stay consistent.

Regular Assessments: Schedule periodic assessments of your fitness levels. This can include measurements like heart rate, flexibility tests, or timed walks. Comparing these assessments over time offers a clear picture of your progress and areas that may need more focus.

Celebrate Milestones: Acknowledge and celebrate your achievements. Whether it's reaching a specific number of workout sessions or achieving a particular goal, reward yourself for your hard work. Positive reinforcement enhances motivation and encourages consistency.

Adjust Goals as Needed: Reassess your goals periodically. If you find a goal too easy or too challenging, modify it accordingly. Your fitness journey is dynamic, and adjusting goals ensures they remain challenging yet achievable.

Seek Professional Guidance: Consider consulting a fitness trainer or physical therapist, especially if you have specific health concerns. They can help you set realistic goals, design a tailored workout plan, and monitor your progress effectively.

By setting achievable goals and diligently tracking your progress, you'll not only stay motivated but also maintain consistency in your senior workout routine. Remember, progress might be gradual, but every step forward is a significant accomplishment toward a healthier and more active lifestyle.

Incorporating social activities and group exercises for motivation

Incorporating social activities and group exercises into a senior fitness routine can significantly enhance motivation, making the journey towards health and wellness both enjoyable and fulfilling. Here's how you can create a supportive and engaging environment for seniors through social interactions and group exercises:

1. Community-Based Classes:

Organize fitness classes specifically tailored for seniors in local community centers or senior living facilities. These classes could include gentle yoga, water aerobics, or tai chi. Group sessions provide a sense of camaraderie and support, encouraging seniors to attend regularly.

2. Walking or Hiking Groups:

Create walking or hiking groups where seniors can explore nature together. Regular outdoor activities not only improve physical health but also offer mental relaxation. Walking and chatting with others make the experience enjoyable and motivate participants to keep coming back.

3. Dance Classes:

Dancing is a fun way to stay active. Arrange dance classes, such as ballroom dancing or line dancing, where seniors can socialize while improving their coordination and fitness. The joy of dancing in a group setting can boost motivation and make exercise more appealing.

4. Social Fitness Events:

Host social fitness events like fitness fairs or health expos. Invite local fitness instructors and health professionals to conduct workshops and interactive sessions. These events provide opportunities for seniors to learn new exercises, get expert guidance, and socialize with peers who share similar fitness goals.

5. Team Sports:

Introduce low-impact team sports like pickleball, bocce ball, or chair volleyball. These games encourage friendly competition and teamwork, fostering a sense of belonging and motivation to stay active. Team sports also promote social interaction and create a supportive community.

6. Group Challenges:

Organize fitness challenges within the group, such as step-count challenges or mini-marathons. Working towards a common goal instills a sense of achievement and encourages seniors to remain consistent in their efforts. Recognize and celebrate participants' accomplishments to reinforce motivation.

7. Fitness Support Groups:

Establish fitness support groups where seniors can share their experiences, challenges, and successes. Regular meetings create a supportive environment where members can offer encouragement, advice, and motivation to one another. Knowing that others are facing similar challenges can boost morale and commitment to fitness goals.

8. Interactive Workshops and Seminars:

Host interactive workshops on topics like nutrition, mindfulness, or stress management. Seniors can learn valuable information while engaging in discussions with experts and fellow participants. These educational events enhance motivation by emphasizing the holistic approach to well-being.

9. Outdoor Picnics and Exercise Sessions:

Combine physical activity with social gatherings by organizing outdoor picnics followed by light exercise sessions. Enjoying healthy meals together and engaging in group exercises in a relaxed outdoor setting fosters social bonds and keeps participants motivated to maintain their fitness routines.

10. Intergenerational Activities:

Arrange activities that involve interaction with younger generations, such as joint art projects, gardening, or storytelling sessions. The exchange of experiences and energy between seniors and younger individuals can be inspiring, fostering a sense of purpose and motivation among seniors.

Incorporating social activities and group exercises not only promotes physical fitness but also creates a sense of community, support, and motivation among seniors. By fostering connections and making fitness enjoyable, seniors are more likely to stay committed to their exercise routines, leading to improved overall health and well-being.

Overcoming common obstacles and staying consistent with workouts

Regular exercise is vital for seniors' physical and mental well-being. However, staying consistent with workouts can be challenging due to various obstacles. Here's how seniors can overcome common hurdles and maintain a consistent workout routine:

1. Health Concerns:

Solution: Consult a healthcare professional before starting any exercise program. They can provide tailored advice, ensuring workouts are safe and appropriate for individual health conditions.

2. Lack of Motivation:

Solution: Set clear and achievable goals, celebrate small victories, and find an exercise buddy or join group classes to enhance motivation. Incorporate activities you enjoy to make workouts more engaging.

3. Joint Pain and Limited Mobility:

Solution: Opt for low-impact exercises like swimming, cycling, or chair exercises that are gentle on joints. Incorporate flexibility and balance exercises to improve mobility and reduce pain.

4. Fatigue and Low Energy:

Solution: Prioritize sleep, maintain a balanced diet, and stay hydrated to boost energy levels. Consider breaking workouts into shorter sessions throughout the day if fatigue is a concern.

5. Fear of Injury:

Solution: Start with simple exercises and gradually increase intensity. Use proper equipment and techniques, and don't hesitate to seek guidance from fitness professionals to ensure exercises are performed safely.

6. Lack of Time:

Solution: Incorporate short, effective workouts into daily activities. Opt for quick exercises like squats, leg lifts, or brisk walking during television commercials or while waiting for a meal to cook.

7. Weather Constraints:

Solution: Have a backup indoor exercise plan for days when weather conditions prevent outdoor activities. Use online workout videos or invest in home exercise equipment for indoor workouts.

8. Loneliness and Isolation:

Solution: Participate in group exercise classes or social fitness events tailored for seniors. Join community centers or senior clubs where you can engage in group activities, fostering social connections and combating loneliness.

9. Boredom:

Solution: Vary your workouts to keep them interesting. Try different exercises, incorporate outdoor activities, or participate in dancing or sports classes to add excitement and prevent boredom.

10. Lack of Support:

Solution: Communicate your fitness goals with friends and family, seeking their encouragement. Consider finding a workout buddy or joining online fitness communities where you can share experiences and receive support from like-minded individuals.

11. Inconsistent Routine:

Solution: Establish a fixed workout schedule and treat it like an unbreakable appointment. Consistency is key, so make exercise a non-negotiable part of your daily routine.

12. Self-Compassion:

Solution: Be kind to yourself. Understand that setbacks happen, and it's essential to forgive yourself and resume your workout routine without guilt. Consistency is about the long-term effort, not perfection.

By addressing these obstacles with tailored solutions and a positive mindset, seniors can overcome challenges and maintain a consistent workout routine. Regular exercise not only enhances physical health but also boosts mood, energy levels, and overall quality of life, making it well worth the effort.

CHAPTER 6

Nutrition and Recovery

Proper nutrition and adequate recovery play pivotal roles in ensuring seniors derive maximum benefits from their workouts. Here's a guide on how seniors can optimize their nutrition and recovery strategies to support their fitness goals and overall well-being:

1.Balanced Nutrition:

Whole Foods: Focus on a balanced diet rich in whole foods like fruits, vegetables, lean proteins, whole grains, and healthy fats. These provide essential nutrients, vitamins, and minerals necessary for energy and muscle function.

Hydration: Stay well-hydrated before, during, and after workouts.Lack of hydration can result in tiredness and muscle cramps. Seniors should make a point to consume water consistently throughout the day.Protein Intake: Include adequate protein sources such as lean meats, poultry, fish, eggs, dairy, legumes, and nuts. Protein supports muscle repair and growth, crucial for maintaining strength and mobility.

Calcium and Vitamin D: Seniors need sufficient calcium and vitamin D for bone health. Include dairy products, fortified foods, leafy greens, and sunlight exposure to support bone density.

2. Pre-Workout Nutrition:

Carbohydrates: Consume complex carbohydrates like whole grains, fruits, and vegetables before workouts. Carbs provide a readily available energy source, aiding in endurance during exercise.

Light Protein Snack: Pair carbohydrates with a small amount of protein for sustained energy. Examples include a banana with peanut butter or yogurt with granola.

3. Post-Workout Nutrition:

Protein-Rich Snack: Consume a protein-rich snack within an hour after exercising. This could be a protein shake, a small chicken breast, or a handful of almonds. Protein supports muscle recovery and growth.

Rehydration: Replenish fluids lost during the workout. Water, coconut water, or electrolyte-rich drinks can help restore hydration levels.

4. Adequate Rest and Recovery:

Ensure you obtain 7-9 hours of undisturbed sleep nightly. High-quality sleep is essential for both muscle recovery and overall health.

Active Recovery: Engage in light, low-impact activities like walking or gentle stretching on rest days. This promotes blood circulation, reducing muscle stiffness.

Muscle Relaxation: Consider activities like yoga or meditation to relax both the body and mind. These practices enhance flexibility and reduce stress, aiding in overall recovery.

Massage and Foam Rolling: Regular massages or foam rolling sessions can help alleviate muscle soreness and improve flexibility.

5. Listen to Your Body:

Be attentive to persistent pain or discomfort. If you encounter unusual pain, allow yourself adequate rest and seek guidance from a healthcare professional if needed.

Rest Days: Don't overlook the importance of rest days in your workout routine. Overtraining can lead to injuries and burnout. Plan for at least one or two rest days per week.

6. Consultation and Monitoring:

Professional Guidance: If possible, consult a nutritionist or a fitness expert who specializes in senior fitness. They can create a personalized nutrition plan and workout routine tailored to your needs.

Regular Health Check-ups: Regular medical check-ups can help monitor your overall health, ensuring your nutrition and exercise plans align with your specific health requirements.

By incorporating these nutrition and recovery strategies, seniors can enhance the effectiveness of their workouts, promote muscle recovery, and support their overall health and vitality. Remember, a holistic approach to fitness, including proper nutrition and recovery, leads to better results and a higher quality of life.

Importance of a balanced diet and hydration for seniors

The importance of a well-rounded diet and proper hydration for the elderly cannot be overstated. As individuals age, their nutritional needs change, making it essential to maintain a balanced diet and stay well-hydrated to support overall health and well-being.

1. Nutritional Support:

A well-rounded diet provides essential nutrients such as vitamins, minerals, proteins, and fiber that are crucial for maintaining optimal health in seniors. These nutrients support the immune system, bone health, and organ function, promoting longevity and vitality.

2. Energy and Stamina:

Balanced nutrition ensures a steady supply of energy, enabling seniors to stay active and engaged in daily activities. Proper hydration supports bodily functions and helps prevent fatigue, allowing seniors to maintain their stamina throughout the day.

3. Muscle and Bone Health:

Adequate protein intake is vital for preserving muscle mass, strength, and bone density, which tend to decline with age. Calcium and vitamin D, found in many balanced diets, support bone health and reduce the risk of osteoporosis and fractures in the elderly.

4. Disease Prevention:

A well-balanced diet rich in antioxidants, vitamins, and minerals can help prevent chronic diseases such as heart disease, diabetes, and certain cancers. Hydration, on the other hand, supports kidney function and aids in maintaining healthy blood pressure levels, reducing the risk of cardiovascular issues.

5. Cognitive Function:

Specific nutrients like omega-3 fatty acids and antioxidants play a vital role in promoting brain health and cognitive function.A balanced diet that includes these nutrients can help prevent cognitive decline and enhance memory and focus in seniors.

6. Digestive Health:

Fiber-rich foods in a balanced diet promote digestive health, preventing constipation and other gastrointestinal issues commonly experienced by the elderly. Proper hydration also supports healthy digestion and prevents dehydration-related digestive problems.

7. Mood and Emotional Well-being:

Nutritional deficiencies can impact mood and emotional well-being. Consuming a well-rounded diet rich in nutrients supports the production of neurotransmitters, helping to maintain a positive outlook and reduce the risk of depression and anxiety.

8. Faster Recovery:

In case of illness or injury, seniors with a well-rounded diet and proper hydration tend to recover faster. Adequate nutrients and hydration support the body's healing processes, aiding in a quicker recovery and reducing the risk of complications.

In summary, a well-rounded diet and proper hydration are fundamental pillars of senior health. By maintaining a balanced diet and staying adequately hydrated, seniors can enhance their overall quality of life, maintain their independence, and enjoy a healthier and more active lifestyle well into their golden years.

Rest and recovery techniques to prevent fatigue and injuries

As seniors engage in regular exercise routines, it becomes crucial to implement effective rest and recovery techniques to prevent fatigue and injuries. Here are some valuable strategies tailored to the needs of older adults, ensuring they can maintain their fitness levels safely and sustainably.

Adequate Sleep: Seniors should aim for 7-9 hours of sleep each night. Quality sleep is essential for muscle repair, hormone regulation, and overall energy levels. Establishing a consistent sleep schedule can significantly enhance recovery.

Proper Nutrition: Consuming a balanced diet rich in protein, vitamins, and minerals is vital for seniors. Protein aids in muscle repair, while vitamins and minerals support overall bodily functions. Adequate hydration is also crucial to prevent dehydration, especially during and after workouts.

Active Recovery: Engage in low-intensity activities like walking, swimming, or yoga on rest days. These activities enhance blood circulation, reduce muscle stiffness, and promote joint flexibility without putting excessive strain on the body.

Stretching and Flexibility Exercises: Incorporate gentle stretching exercises into your routine. Stretching improves flexibility, reduces muscle tension, and enhances joint mobility. Focus on major muscle groups, holding each stretch for 15-30 seconds without bouncing.

Foam Rolling: Using a foam roller can help release muscle knots and improve blood flow. Seniors can use foam rollers to perform self-myofascial release, which aids in muscle recovery and reduces muscle soreness.

Massage Therapy: Regular massages can be beneficial for seniors. Massage therapy relaxes muscles, reduces inflammation, and promotes overall relaxation. It can also alleviate joint pain and enhance flexibility.

Mind-Body Techniques: Practices like meditation, deep breathing, and mindfulness can reduce stress and promote mental relaxation. Stress management is essential for overall well-being and can contribute significantly to the recovery process.

Listen to Your Body: Seniors should pay close attention to their bodies. If they experience persistent pain, fatigue, or discomfort, it's crucial to allow adequate time for rest and, if necessary, seek medical advice.Persisting despite pain can result in injuries and hindrances.

Consult a Professional: Before starting any exercise regimen, seniors should consult a healthcare provider or a certified fitness trainer who specializes in working with older adults. A tailored workout plan, considering individual health conditions and fitness levels, can significantly reduce the risk of injuries.

Stay Consistent: Consistency is key to effective rest and recovery. Establishing a regular exercise routine and adhering to proper rest and recovery techniques will not only prevent fatigue and injuries but also improve overall fitness and quality of life.

By incorporating these rest and recovery techniques into their fitness regimen, seniors can enjoy the benefits of exercise while minimizing the risk of fatigue and injuries, ensuring a healthier and more active lifestyle in the long run.

Incorporating proper nutrition to support exercise and promote muscle recovery

Incorporating Adequate Nutrition to Support Exercise and Enhance Muscle Recovery in Seniors

Proper nutrition plays a pivotal role in supporting exercise routines and promoting muscle recovery, especially for seniors. Here are essential guidelines tailored to the nutritional needs of older adults, ensuring they can maintain their physical health and vitality:

Balanced Diet: Seniors should focus on consuming a well-balanced diet that includes a variety of whole foods. This should encompass lean proteins, such as poultry, fish, beans, and tofu, which aid in muscle repair and growth. Incorporating whole grains, fruits, vegetables, and healthy fats like avocados and nuts provides essential vitamins, minerals, and fiber necessary for overall health.

Protein Intake: Adequate protein intake is crucial for seniors to support muscle recovery and prevent muscle loss, a common concern with aging. Including protein-rich foods in every meal can enhance muscle repair and maintenance. Sources like lean meats, eggs, dairy products, and plant-based options like legumes and quinoa are excellent choices.

Hydration: Proper hydration is vital during and after exercise. Seniors should drink water regularly throughout the day, especially before, during, and after workouts. Dehydration can impair muscle function and delay recovery, so it's essential to maintain adequate fluid levels.

Micronutrients: Seniors should focus on micronutrients like vitamins and minerals, which are essential for various bodily functions. Calcium and vitamin D are crucial for bone health, while vitamins C and E possess antioxidant properties, aiding in reducing exercise-induced oxidative stress. A diverse diet including colorful fruits and vegetables ensures a wide range of essential nutrients.

Omega-3 Fatty Acids: Incorporating sources of omega-3 fatty acids, such as fatty fish (like salmon and mackerel), flaxseeds, and walnuts, can reduce inflammation and support joint health, essential for seniors engaging in physical activities.

Timing of Meals: Seniors should consider timing their meals around their exercise routines. Consuming a balanced meal or snack containing protein and carbohydrates within an hour after exercising can facilitate muscle recovery and replenish glycogen stores.

Limit Processed Foods: Minimize the intake of processed foods, sugary snacks, and excessive sodium, as these can contribute to inflammation and negatively impact overall health. Instead, opt for whole, unprocessed foods to provide the body with essential nutrients without added unhealthy components.

Consult a Nutritionist: Seniors with specific dietary concerns or health conditions should consult a registered dietitian or nutritionist. These professionals can create personalized nutrition plans, addressing individual needs and ensuring seniors receive the right balance of nutrients to support their exercise routines and muscle recovery.

By incorporating these nutritional strategies, seniors can enhance their exercise performance, support muscle recovery, and maintain overall health and well-being as they age, enabling them to enjoy an active and fulfilling lifestyle.

CHAPTER 7

<u>**Dealing with Challenges**</u>

Staying active is crucial for seniors to maintain their overall health and mobility. However, aging bodies can present certain challenges during workouts. Here are some common issues seniors might face and effective ways to address them:

Joint Pain and Arthritis: Arthritis and joint pain are prevalent among seniors, making movement uncomfortable. Low-impact exercises such as swimming, walking, or cycling can be gentler on the joints. Additionally, proper warm-up and cool-down routines, along with joint-friendly activities like yoga, can help alleviate discomfort.

Reduced Balance: Seniors often experience a decline in balance, increasing the risk of falls during workouts. Incorporating balance exercises into the routine, such as standing on one leg or using stability balls, can help improve balance and stability. It's also advisable to work out near a sturdy surface or have a chair nearby for support.

Muscle Weakness: Muscle weakness is a natural part of aging, but resistance training exercises using light weights or resistance bands can help build muscle strength. Focus on different muscle groups and start with light resistance, gradually increasing it as strength improves.

Chronic Health Conditions: Seniors may have chronic health conditions like diabetes, heart disease, or hypertension, which require careful management during workouts. Consulting healthcare providers and fitness professionals who specialize in senior fitness is essential. They can design tailored workout plans considering these conditions and monitor the exercises to ensure safety.

Low Energy Levels: Aging bodies might have lower energy levels. Seniors can combat fatigue by ensuring they get adequate sleep, stay hydrated, and maintain a balanced diet. Listening to their bodies and allowing for rest days when necessary is equally important. Engaging in social or group exercises can also boost motivation and energy levels.

Fear of Injury: Seniors may fear getting injured during workouts, which can discourage them from staying active. Working with a certified trainer experienced in senior fitness can provide reassurance. They can guide seniors through exercises with proper form, ensuring safety and preventing injuries.

Cognitive Challenges: Cognitive decline can affect a senior's ability to follow workout routines. Simple, repetitive exercises with clear instructions can be helpful. Additionally, incorporating activities that challenge the mind, such as dance or certain sports, can enhance cognitive function while keeping workouts engaging.

Lack of Motivation: Maintaining motivation can be challenging, especially when progress is slow. Setting realistic goals, celebrating small achievements, and varying workout routines can keep seniors motivated. Engaging in social activities or finding a workout buddy can also provide the necessary encouragement and accountability.

By addressing these challenges with patience, tailored exercise routines, and professional guidance, seniors can overcome obstacles and continue to enjoy the numerous physical and mental benefits of regular exercise, leading to a healthier and more fulfilling lifestyle.

Addressing fear and anxiety related to exercise

It's natural for seniors to experience fear and anxiety related to exercise, especially if they have concerns about safety, physical limitations, or past injuries. Overcoming these fears is crucial to maintain a healthy and active lifestyle. Here are some effective strategies to address fear and anxiety during workouts for seniors:

Education and Awareness: Providing seniors with information about the benefits of exercise, along with the reassurance that many others face similar fears, can be empowering. Understanding the positive impact of physical activity on overall health, mobility, and mood can alleviate anxiety.

Start Slow and Gradual: Encourage seniors to start with gentle, low-impact exercises. Beginning with activities like walking, stretching, or chair exercises allows them to build confidence and gradually increase the intensity as they feel more comfortable. Slow progress is still progress.

Professional Guidance: Working with certified trainers or physical therapists who specialize in senior fitness can provide seniors with a sense of security. These professionals can create personalized exercise plans tailored to individual needs and limitations, ensuring safe and effective workouts.

Social Support: Exercising in a supportive and social environment can significantly reduce anxiety. Encourage seniors to participate in group fitness classes, community exercise programs, or find a workout buddy. The camaraderie and encouragement from peers can boost confidence and alleviate fears.

Mind-Body Techniques: Introducing relaxation techniques such as deep breathing, meditation, or yoga can help seniors manage anxiety. These practices not only promote physical relaxation but also enhance mental well-being, reducing overall stress and fear related to exercise.

Positive Reinforcement: Celebrate small achievements and milestones. Positive reinforcement can boost self-confidence and motivate seniors to continue their exercise routines.Motivate them to concentrate on improvement rather than aiming for flawless outcomes.

Familiar Environment: Seniors may feel more comfortable exercising in familiar surroundings. Encourage home-based workouts or exercises in local parks, where they feel at ease. Feeling secure in the environment can significantly reduce anxiety levels.

Setting Realistic Goals: Help seniors set achievable and realistic goals. Dividing complex fitness objectives into smaller, achievable tasks can reduce the feeling of being overwhelmed.Accomplishing these smaller goals provides a sense of accomplishment and boosts confidence.

Regular Communication: Maintain open communication with seniors, addressing their concerns and fears. Encourage them to express their feelings, and be supportive and empathetic. Knowing that their concerns are heard and understood can ease anxiety.

Patience and Encouragement: Seniors may need time to overcome their fears. Patience, encouragement, and a positive attitude can go a long way. Remind them that it's never too late to start and that every effort they make toward staying active is a significant achievement.

By implementing these strategies, seniors can gradually overcome their fears and anxieties related to exercise. With the right support, guidance, and understanding, they can embrace physical activity, leading to improved overall health, confidence, and a greater sense of well-being.

Coping with pain, discomfort, or fatigue during workouts

Experiencing pain, discomfort, or fatigue during workouts is not uncommon, especially for seniors. It's essential to address these sensations appropriately to ensure a safe and effective exercise routine. Here are some strategies to help seniors cope with these challenges:

Listen to Your Body: Seniors need to be mindful of their body's signals while exercising. If they encounter sharp pain, extreme discomfort, or unusual fatigue, it is crucial to cease the activity right away. Continuing despite severe pain can result in injuries.

Modify Exercises: Seniors can modify exercises to suit their comfort levels. For instance, they can perform seated versions of exercises, use lighter weights, or reduce the range of motion. Modifying workouts can help minimize discomfort while still engaging in physical activity.

Warming up and cooling down properly are vital. Gentle warm-up exercises boost blood circulation to the muscles,preparing them for activity and reducing the risk of injury. Cooling down with stretching exercises can help prevent muscle stiffness and enhance flexibility, promoting faster recovery.

Pacing: Seniors should pace themselves during workouts. It's important not to overexert. Encourage them to take breaks between exercises and listen to their bodies' signals of fatigue. Setting a comfortable pace ensures that they can complete the workout without excessive strain.

Stay Hydrated: Dehydration can intensify feelings of fatigue and discomfort. Seniors should drink water before, during, and after exercise to stay properly hydrated. Proper hydration supports overall bodily functions and helps prevent muscle cramps.

Breathing Techniques: Proper breathing techniques can enhance endurance and reduce fatigue. Seniors should focus on deep, rhythmic breathing during exercises. Inhaling and exhaling steadily can help oxygenate the muscles and reduce feelings of breathlessness and fatigue.

Rest and recovery are essential components. Seniors need to give their bodies sufficient time to recover and rejuvenate.between workout sessions. Scheduling regular rest days into their exercise routine ensures muscles have time to repair, reducing the risk of overuse injuries and fatigue.

Seek Professional Guidance: Seniors can benefit from working with certified fitness trainers or physical therapists, especially those experienced in senior fitness. These professionals can design customized exercise plans, taking into account individual limitations and ensuring seniors engage in safe and appropriate workouts.

Pain Management Techniques: For chronic conditions causing pain, seniors can explore pain management techniques such as gentle massage, heat therapy, or cold packs. Consulting healthcare providers for appropriate pain management strategies is important to address underlying issues.

Rest and recuperation are essential. Seniors should give their bodies the necessary time to recover.. Celebrate achievements, no matter how small, and maintain a positive attitude toward exercise. A positive mindset can help seniors cope better with discomfort and fatigue, motivating them to stay active.

By applying these coping strategies, seniors can engage in regular exercise routines more comfortably, promoting their overall well-being and ensuring a safer and more enjoyable workout experience.

Seeking support and encouragement from family, friends, or support groups

Seeking Support and Encouragement from Loved Ones and Support Groups for Senior Workouts

Engaging in regular physical activity can be significantly enhanced when seniors receive support and encouragement from their family, friends, and support groups. Here's how the encouragement from these sources can positively impact seniors' workout routines:

Emotional Support: Family and friends can provide emotional encouragement, creating a positive atmosphere that motivates seniors to stay active. Knowing that their loved ones support their fitness journey boosts seniors' confidence and commitment to exercise.

Accountability: When seniors share their fitness goals with family or friends, they establish a sense of accountability. Loved ones can check in on their progress, celebrate achievements, and gently remind them to stay consistent. This accountability can help seniors stay on track with their workout routines.

Companionship: Exercising with friends or family members can turn workouts into enjoyable social activities. Seniors can join group fitness classes or take walks together, making the experience more engaging and fun. Having companions provides motivation and reduces feelings of isolation during exercise.

Encouragement for Progress: Celebrating even small milestones and achievements can boost seniors' confidence. Family and friends can offer praise and encouragement for every step forward, reinforcing the idea that their efforts are valued and worthwhile.

Knowledge and Advice: Family and friends can share their knowledge about exercise routines, healthy habits, and nutrition. They can provide valuable advice on effective workouts or suggest activities that align with seniors' interests and physical abilities.

Support Groups: Support groups specifically designed for seniors can offer a sense of community and understanding. Interacting with peers who face similar challenges and goals can provide a unique form of encouragement. Sharing experiences, successes, and struggles within these groups can foster a sense of belonging and motivation.

Flexibility and Adaptation: Loved ones can support seniors by being flexible and adaptive to their needs. Understanding that physical abilities might change over time, family and friends can help modify activities, ensuring they remain safe and enjoyable.

Celebrating Efforts: Recognizing seniors' commitment to their fitness goals, regardless of the outcome, is crucial. Celebrating their efforts, dedication, and consistency reinforces the importance of staying active and encourages them to keep going, even on challenging days.

In summary, the encouragement and support from family, friends, and support groups create a strong foundation for seniors to maintain regular exercise routines. These positive interactions not only enhance physical well-being but also contribute significantly to seniors' emotional and social fulfillment, promoting a healthier and happier lifestyle.

CHAPTER 8

Special Considerations

When seniors engage in exercise routines, there are specific considerations to ensure their safety, well-being, and overall enjoyment. Tailoring workouts to address the unique needs of older adults is essential. Here are some special considerations to keep in mind during senior workouts:

Health Assessment: Before starting any exercise program, seniors should undergo a health assessment by a healthcare provider. This assessment helps identify existing health conditions, limitations, and potential risks. It provides valuable information for designing a personalized and safe workout plan.

Low-Impact Exercises: Seniors should focus on low-impact exercises to reduce stress on joints and minimize the risk of injuries. Activities like walking, swimming, cycling, and chair exercises are gentle on the joints while providing excellent cardiovascular benefits.

Balance and Stability: Balance exercises are crucial for seniors, as they help prevent falls and improve stability. Incorporating exercises that challenge balance, such as standing on one leg or using balance boards, can enhance coordination and prevent accidents.

Flexibility and Stretching: Regular stretching exercises improve flexibility and joint range of motion. Seniors should include dynamic and static stretches in their routine to enhance mobility and reduce muscle stiffness. Flexibility exercises are particularly vital for seniors to maintain their independence and perform daily activities comfortably.

Strength training workouts are vital for preserving muscle mass, bone density, and overall physical strength.Seniors should incorporate resistance exercises using light weights, resistance bands, or bodyweight to improve muscle tone and functional abilities.

Proper Form and Technique: Ensuring seniors use proper form and technique during exercises is crucial to prevent injuries. Working with certified trainers who specialize in senior fitness can provide valuable guidance on correct posture and movements, ensuring safe and effective workouts.

Monitoring Intensity: Seniors should monitor the intensity of their workouts to avoid overexertion. Paying attention to their heart rate, breathing, and overall comfort level can help them adjust the intensity accordingly. It's important to find a balance that challenges them without causing excessive fatigue.

Hydration and Nutrition: Staying hydrated before, during, and after workouts is vital, especially for seniors. Proper nutrition, including a balanced diet rich in nutrients, supports energy levels and overall health. Seniors should consume water and balanced meals to fuel their bodies for exercise and aid in recovery.

Regular Rest and Recovery: Seniors require adequate time for rest and recovery between workout sessions. Proper sleep, along with rest days, allows muscles to repair and prevents overuse injuries. Encouraging seniors to prioritize rest contributes significantly to their overall well-being.

Medical Supervision: For seniors with specific health conditions or chronic illnesses, exercising under medical supervision is crucial. Healthcare providers can offer personalized recommendations and monitor progress, ensuring that the workouts align with the individual's health needs and limitations.

By taking these special considerations into account, seniors can enjoy the numerous benefits of exercise while minimizing the risk of injuries and enhancing their overall quality of life.

Exercise guidelines for seniors with specific health conditions (e.g., arthritis, osteoporosis)

Seniors with specific health conditions like arthritis and osteoporosis can benefit greatly from tailored exercise routines that address their unique needs and limitations. Here are some guidelines to consider when designing workouts for seniors with these conditions:

1. Arthritis:

Low-Impact Exercises: Focus on low-impact activities such as swimming, walking, or stationary cycling to minimize stress on joints. Water aerobics can be particularly beneficial due to its gentle nature and buoyancy.

Range of Motion Exercises: Include exercises that promote joint flexibility and range of motion. Gentle stretching and yoga can help improve mobility and reduce stiffness in arthritic joints.

Strength Training: Incorporate light resistance exercises to strengthen the muscles around affected joints. Start with low weights or resistance bands and gradually increase intensity based on individual comfort levels.

Warm-Up and Cool Down: Begin each session with a thorough warm-up to prepare joints and muscles for activity. Cooling down with stretching exercises can help prevent post-exercise stiffness.

Pain Management: Encourage seniors to manage pain with techniques like heat or cold therapy, as well as over-the-counter pain relief creams. Consulting healthcare providers for suitable pain management strategies is essential.

2. Osteoporosis:

Weight-Bearing Exercises: Engage in weight-bearing exercises such as walking, dancing, or stair climbing to improve bone density. These activities put mild stress on bones, stimulating them to become denser and stronger.

Strength Training: Focus on resistance exercises to target major muscle groups. Using light weights or resistance bands, seniors can enhance muscle strength, which indirectly supports bone health.

Balance and Posture: Include exercises that improve balance and posture, reducing the risk of falls and fractures. Balance exercises like standing on one leg and practicing tai chi can enhance stability.

Avoid High-Impact Activities: Seniors with osteoporosis should avoid high-impact activities that may increase the risk of fractures, such as running or jumping. Instead, opt for low-impact alternatives that provide similar cardiovascular benefits.

Consultation with Healthcare Providers: Seniors with osteoporosis should consult healthcare providers before starting any exercise program. Healthcare professionals can offer guidance on safe activities and recommend appropriate precautions.

<u>**General Tips for Both Conditions:**</u>

Individualized Approach: Tailor exercise programs based on individual abilities, limitations, and comfort levels. What works for one person may not be suitable for another, so personalized plans are crucial.

Regular Monitoring: Regularly assess progress and make adjustments to the exercise routine as needed. Seniors should communicate any discomfort or changes in their condition to healthcare providers and fitness professionals.

Consistency: Encourage seniors to maintain a consistent exercise schedule. Regular, moderate activity provides the most significant benefits for joint health, bone density, and overall well-being.

By following these guidelines and taking a personalized approach, seniors with conditions like arthritis and osteoporosis can engage in safe and effective exercise routines, improving their quality of life and promoting better health outcomes.

Senior-friendly modifications for home workouts and gym environments

Adapting workouts to cater to the needs of seniors is essential for their safety and enjoyment. Here are some senior-friendly modifications for both home workouts and gym environments:

1. Home Workouts:

Chair Exercises: Incorporate seated exercises using a sturdy chair for support. Chair squats, seated leg lifts, and seated marching are excellent options for building strength without putting excessive strain on joints.

Low-Impact Cardio: Choose low-impact cardio exercises like walking in place, marching, or low-impact aerobics to maintain cardiovascular health. These exercises provide a good workout while being gentle on joints.

Bodyweight Strength Training: Use bodyweight exercises like wall push-ups, bodyweight squats, and modified planks. These exercises improve muscle strength and can be adjusted to accommodate varying fitness levels.

Resistance Bands: Integrate resistance bands into workouts to add resistance for strength training exercises. They are versatile, affordable, and offer adjustable resistance levels suitable for seniors.

Home Safety: Ensure a safe environment by removing obstacles, using non-slip mats, and having proper lighting. Seniors should wear supportive footwear to prevent falls during exercises.

2. Gym Environments:

Personal Trainer Guidance: Working with a certified trainer experienced in senior fitness can provide tailored exercise plans. Trainers can assist with proper form, modify exercises, and ensure seniors use equipment safely.

Machine Modifications: Opt for resistance machines with adjustable settings to control resistance levels.Begin with lighter weights and, as strength progresses, gradually increase the weight. Alternatively, opt for resistance bands over machines for a workout that's safer.
Balance and Stability Equipment: Utilize stability balls, balance pads, and wobble boards to enhance balance and stability. These tools help strengthen core muscles and improve overall stability, reducing the risk of falls.

Group Classes: Participate in senior-friendly group fitness classes such as water aerobics, yoga, or tai chi. These classes often cater to varying fitness levels and provide a supportive, social environment.

Access to Amenities: Choose gyms with senior-friendly amenities such as grab bars in changing rooms, well-maintained and well-lit pathways, and accessible facilities. Easy access to water stations and restroom facilities is also important.

Hydration and Rest: Encourage seniors to stay hydrated during workouts and take regular breaks. Overexertion can lead to fatigue, making hydration and rest essential for a safe and enjoyable experience.

By implementing these modifications, both home workouts and gym environments can be transformed into safe, accessible, and enjoyable spaces for seniors to stay active and maintain their overall health and well-being.

<u>**Travel-friendly exercises for seniors who are frequently on the move**</u>

Staying active while traveling is important for seniors, and there are plenty of exercises that can be done on the go without the need for specialized equipment. Here are some travel-friendly exercises tailored for seniors who are frequently on the move:

1. Walking: Walking is one of the simplest yet effective exercises. Seniors can explore new places by taking leisurely walks. Whether it's around a park, beach, or city streets, walking helps maintain cardiovascular health and keeps the joints flexible.

2. Bodyweight Exercises:

Bodyweight Squats: Stand with feet shoulder-width apart and lower into a squat position. Hold onto a stable surface if needed for balance.

Seated Leg Lifts: Sit on a chair, straighten one or both legs, and hold in place for a few seconds.Lower the leg(s) without allowing the feet to make contact with the ground.Repeat on the other side.

Standing Calf Raises: Stand on a flat surface and rise onto the balls of the feet, then lower the heels back down.This activity enhances calf muscle strength and boosts stability.

3. Resistance Band Exercises: Lightweight and portable, resistance bands are perfect for travelers. They offer various levels of resistance and can be used for a range of exercises targeting different muscle groups, such as bicep curls, shoulder presses, or leg lifts.

4. Yoga and Stretching:

Chair Yoga: Seniors can perform modified yoga poses while sitting on a chair. These activities enhance flexibility, and balance, and promote relaxation.

Stretching: Incorporate gentle stretching exercises targeting major muscle groups. Stretching helps maintain flexibility and reduces muscle stiffness.

5. Water Workouts: If traveling near a pool or beach, water exercises are excellent for seniors. Water provides resistance, making movements effective yet gentle on the joints. Water aerobics, walking in water, or simple leg lifts in the pool are great options.

6. Fitness Apps and Online Videos: Seniors can access fitness apps and online videos designed for travelers. These resources offer guided workouts ranging from seated exercises to light aerobics, providing convenient exercise options right in their accommodation.

7. Stair Climbing: If staying in a multi-story building, seniors can use stairs for a low-impact cardiovascular workout. Climbing stairs helps strengthen leg muscles and improves cardiovascular health.

8. Dance: Put on some music and dance! Dancing is not only enjoyable but also a great way to stay active. Seniors can dance to their favorite tunes in the comfort of their hotel room or accommodation.

These travel-friendly exercises allow seniors to maintain their fitness routines, improve flexibility, and enhance overall well-being while on the move. Staying active during travels not only supports physical health but also adds enjoyment and vitality to their experiences away from home.

Conclusion

Encouragement for seniors to embrace the benefits of regular exercise

Dear Seniors,

We understand that staying active might seem challenging, but it's important to recognize the incredible benefits that regular exercise can bring to your life. By incorporating physical activity into your routine, you're not just enhancing your physical health; you're investing in your overall well-being and happiness. Here's some encouragement to help you embrace the wonders of staying active:

Improved Health: Regular exercise strengthens your heart, boosts your immune system, and helps manage chronic conditions. It's a powerful tool in maintaining good health, allowing you to enjoy life to the fullest.

Increased Energy: Believe it or not, staying active can actually increase your energy levels. Engaging in regular physical activity enhances stamina, making everyday tasks easier and more enjoyable.

Enhanced Mobility: Exercise keeps your muscles and joints flexible, improving your range of motion. This increased mobility ensures you can maintain your independence and move with ease.

Emotional Wellness: Engaging in physical activities is associated with enhanced mental well-being.It reduces stress, anxiety, and depression, providing a natural mood boost. Regular exercise stimulates the release of endorphins, the "feel-good" hormones, leaving you with a sense of accomplishment and contentment.

Social Connections: Participating in group classes or exercise activities can be a wonderful way to meet new people and strengthen existing relationships. Sharing your fitness journey with others creates a supportive and uplifting community.

Quality Sleep: Exercise contributes to better sleep quality. A good night's rest is essential for overall health, and regular physical activity helps you achieve that much-needed restorative sleep.

Boosted Confidence: Achieving your fitness goals, no matter how small they may seem, boosts your self-esteem and confidence. Embracing physical challenges and overcoming them empowers you in various aspects of life.

Longevity: Studies show that regular exercise is linked to a longer lifespan. By staying active, you're investing in a healthier, happier, and longer life surrounded by the people you love.

Remember, it's never too late to start. Every step you take, every stretch you do, and every moment of physical activity matters. Find activities you enjoy, whether it's dancing, walking, swimming, or yoga, and make them a part of your routine.

Your well-being is worth the effort, and the benefits of regular exercise will enrich your life in ways you might not even imagine. So, lace up your shoes, put on your favorite workout attire, and let's embrace this journey together. Here's to your health, happiness, and the countless joys that regular exercise can bring into your life!

Resources and references for further information and support

National Institute on Aging (NIA) - Go4Life: The NIA's Go4Life campaign offers free resources, exercise videos, and tips specifically designed for seniors. Visit their website for workout plans, instructional videos, and motivational content: Go4Life

AARP Fitness and Exercise: AARP provides a wide range of articles, videos, and expert advice on senior fitness and exercise. Their website covers various topics, from low-impact workouts to nutrition tips: AARP Fitness

SilverSneakers: SilverSneakers is a popular senior fitness program available at many gyms and community centers. Their website offers workout routines, nutrition guidance, and social connections for seniors: SilverSneakers

American Council on Exercise (ACE): ACE provides valuable resources on senior fitness, including articles, workout guides, and expert advice. Visit their site for evidence-based information and exercise ideas: ACE Senior Fitness

Centers for Disease Control and Prevention (CDC) - Physical Activity for Older Adults: The CDC offers guidelines, resources, and research-based information on physical activity for older adults.

Access their resources to learn about the importance of staying active as you age: CDC Older Adults

Local Community Centers and Senior Centers: Many local community centers and senior centers offer fitness classes tailored to seniors. Check with your local facilities for in-person or virtual classes, as well as resources specific to your community.

YouTube: YouTube is a treasure trove of workout videos for seniors. Many fitness trainers and organizations upload exercise routines catering to various fitness levels and health conditions. Search for terms like "senior fitness" or "senior workout" to find suitable videos.

Fitness Apps: There are several fitness apps designed for seniors, offering customized workout plans and tracking features. Look for apps with high ratings and positive reviews on app stores, and choose one that suits your preferences and goals.

Remember, before starting any new exercise program, it's advisable to consult your healthcare provider, especially if you have underlying health conditions or concerns. They can provide personalized recommendations and ensure your safety as you embark on your fitness journey.

THANK YOU FOR READING!

9 798867 251345